Dr. Sebi: 100% Natural Remedy 4 Female Reproductive System Disorders!

Steps On How To Use Dr. Sebi Methodology To Treat & Reverse The Root-Cause Of: Fibroids, Infertility, Endometriosis, Abnormal Uterine Bleeding, PCOS, POI, Cervical Cancer & Interstitial Cystitis Without Surgery.

Clement Jacob

Copyright Notice. By Clement Jacob

Table of Contents

Introduction

Have you been trying so hard to get pregnant and become a mother that you have spent too much money buying and consuming of ineffective and very expensive supplement and drugs to treat infertility and other form of female reproductive system disorder without getting your desired result?

Have you been to various hospitals that you have been written off by medical doctors, family members and friends that you are barren and can't be a mother because you are suffering from either: fibroids, infertility, endometriosis, abnormal uterine bleeding, PCOS, POI, cervical cancer, interstitial cystitis etc. that you desire to prove them wrong by getting pregnant?

Are you finding it difficult to get and keep pregnancy because of countless miscarriage that you have suffered in the past and you are gradually getting to the age of menopause?

Do you desire a 100% natural remedy to cleanse/detox your entire body system through an intra-cellular level to get rid of the root-cause of female reproductive system disorder and revitalized your body system to become pregnant and be the mother you have always dream of?

Do you desire a healthy life, free from disease and other forms of female reproductive system disorders?

If your answer to any of the question above is YES, thank goodness because you are at the right place and will soon be declared **FERTILE** by the same doctors who declared you "barren".

However, in this guide, Clement Jacob will expose you on how to use late Dr. Sebi 2 steps of healings methodology, alkaline diets and herbs to cleanse your entire body system, treat and reverse the root-cause of female reproductive system disorders like fibroids, infertility, endometriosis, abnormal uterine bleeding, PCOS, POI, cervical cancer, interstitial cystitis etc. to make you become pregnant and be a mother that you have always wanted to be.

CHAPTER ONE
Female Reproductive System Review
What is Female Reproductive System?

When talking about female reproductive system, we will need to talk about what reproduction is all about first. So, what is reproduction? Reproduction is the process by which living things produced their own kind or young ones for continuity or making sure the specie is kept alive. However, all the organs that functions together to reproduced are what made up the reproductive system.

What Are the Components of the Female Reproductive System?

The female reproductive system is made of some components known as:

1. The Vulva: the vulva is the external part of the female reproductive organ that helps to covers vagina's opening and other reproductive organs of female.

2. The Mons pubis: the Mons pubis is the fleshy area that is at the top of the vagina.

12

3. The Labia: The labia are just like the lips. It's the 2 pairs of skin flaps that surround the vaginal.

4. The Clitoris: the clitoris is a small sensory organ that is at the point where the labia meet at the front of the vulva.

5. Vagina: the vagina is a hollow muscular tube that its opening is partially covered by a skin like tissue called 'hymen' and it can expand and contract and extends to the uterus from its opening. The muscular walls in the vagina are lined with mucous membrane that helps to moist and protect it. T
However, the vagina has three basic functions that it performs which include:

   i.   It is an opening where penis penetrates during sexual activities or intercourse.

   ii.   It serves as a pathway through which women give birth or reproduced.

   iii.   Finally, it is the pathway though which the menstrual blood flow out of the body.

6. The Cervix: the cervix has a thick and strong wall with a small opening but widen during child's birth.

However, the cervix is the point where the vagina and the uterus connect.

7. The Uterus: the uterus has an upside-down pear shape with strong muscular walls (the muscle have the potency to expand and contract as it accommodates a developing fetus and to push out the baby at the point of delivery (labor)) and thick lining.

8. The Fallopian tubes: the fallopian tube is connected to the ovaries and the uterus at the upper Conner of the uterus.

9. The Ovaries: the ovaries are two oval-shaped organs that produces, store and release egg cells (ova) into the fallopian tubes (ovulation). They are also, part of the endocrine system as they produces both estrogen and progesterone hormone which are female sex hormone. This two ova-shaped organs are located at the upper left and right side of the uterus

How the Female Reproductive System Works?

The female reproductive system consists of several organs

which makes it to perform some certain functions. First and foremost, the ovary helps to produce the ova known as "oocytes or egg cells" However, the egg cells (ova) will then be transported to the point where it can be fertilized known as "Fallopian tube". Once the egg cells have been transported to the fallopian tube, the woman will need to be inseminated or engage in a sexual activities or intercourse for the man to release the sperm which will be release through the vagina and transported through the cervix and uterus to the fallopian tube where the egg cells will be fertilized. Once the ova have been fertilized, it will now be transported to the uterus (home for the fetus) and the reproductive cycle hormones will be secreted to thickened the uterine lining and the fertilized ova will then be implanted to the thickened uterine lining and will keep developing. Once the fertilized egg is implanted, there won't be any menstrual period again but if eventually, it does not implant, the uterine lining will be flush out as menstrual period. Finally, the fertilized eggs will develop to become a child. Eventually, the woman will give birth.

However, women that are in their menopause stage, their

reproductive system will stop producing the reproductive hormones needed for the reproductive cycle and their menstrual period will become irregular and eventually stop. If after a year, the menstrual period stop showing up, it means that, the woman is considered to be menopausal.

What are The Types of Female Reproductive Disorders?

There are various types of female reproductive disorder, but I am going to center on the most common ones. They include: uterine fibroids,

1. Uterine Fibroids: Uterine fibroid is the most common female reproductive disorder that is non-cancerous tumors that usually affect women that are in their child bearing age. Within this age, some women might experience some growth of muscle cells or tissues in or around the wall of their womb and sometimes, both in the wall of their womb or uterus. Although there is nothing to be traced as the causes of uterine fibroids but there are some certain risk factors that researchers believe can increase the

risk of having uterine fibroid. These risk factors include: being black (African-American) and obesity or excess weight gain.

However, these types of female reproductive disorder have some symptoms which include:

i.   Constant urination

ii.   Experience some sort of pain during sexual intercourse.

iii.   The lower abdomen will always look full.

iv.   Bleeding between period or might be experiencing heavy pain during menstruation.

v.   Experience lower back pain.

vi.   Multiple miscarriage and some times, early labor.

vii.   Infertility (might not conceive at all)

2. Infertility is the inability to become pregnant after having unprotected sexual intercourse for a long period of time (one year or more).

    This issue of infertility is not only linked to women but it's general and common to both men and women. However, there are lots of organs that comes together to made up the female reproductive system in which if one of the organ malfunctions, it can lead to infertility. So, the causes of infertility include: untreated gonorrhea or chlamydia, PCOS, hypothalamus and pituitary glands disorder, fibroid, blocked fallopian tube, ovaries malfunctioning, poor quality eggs, endometriosis etc.

3. Polycystic Ovary Syndrome (PCOS): this type of female reproductive system disorder happens as a result of hormone imbalance where their adrenal gland and ovaries produces more of male hormone than the normal amount it's supposed to produce. However, this disorder is common to women at the age of childbearing and women that are overweight that cyst (fluid-filled sacs) tend to develop on their ovaries making it to malfunction and once they begin to suffer from this reproductive disorder, their risk of getting or suffering from diabetes and heart diseases will increase. Till date there is no cause of this type of disorder but since it is basically caused by hormone imbalance, I can categorically say that,

genes, insulin resistance and inflammation can be a risk factor for PCOS.

However, certain symptoms to experience by people suffering from PCOS include:

i.   Infertility (unable to conceive or get pregnant)

ii.   More of male features such as too much hair growth on the chest, toes or thumbs and the face.

iii.   Head hair may become thinning or get bald.

iv.   Frequent pelvic pain.

v.   Skin might have some patches of thick dark brown or possibly black.

vi.   The skin will always be oily

vii.   Acne or dandruff might begin to show up.

Please note that, you might not experience all this symptoms but if you experience at least two of it, then it's advisable to confirm if you are suffering from PCOS before knowing the next line of action.

4. Endometriosis: this type of female reproductive system disorder happen when the tissues that is made to lines the womb or uterus, grow and

developed elsewhere (on the bowel, ovaries, bladder or behind the uterus). Don't forget that the uterus is the home for the fetus in which if the tissues grow elsewhere instead of the uterus, it will end up leading to some health challenges.

However, symptoms that are link to endometriosis include:

i.   Infertility (unable to conceive get pregnant)

ii.   Menstruation (period) are usually heavy.

iii.   Experience pelvic, lower back or abdomen pain.

Please note that some women do not show any symptoms but will find it almost impossible to get pregnant.

5. Cervical cancer: this type of female reproductive system disorder is very common to women of childbearing age and it is caused by human papillomavirus (HPV). Research shows that, this type of female reproductive disorder affect more than 11,000 women (mostly women at the age of childbearing) yearly. Although, there are medical

treatment for cervical cancer but it treatment can lead to infertility that is where Dr. Sebi methodology come in play.

However, the symptoms for cervical cancer include:

i. Heavy bleeding during period.

ii. Excessive bleeding during and after sex.

iii. Unnecessary pain and discomfort during sexual intercourse.

iv. Unpleasant vagina discharge.

v. Pelvis or lower back pain

6. Primary Ovarian Insufficiency (POI): this type of female reproductive system disorder happens to women that are below 40. It makes the ovaries to malfunctions thereby causing irregular period or no period at all, swing mood, pain during sex, hot flashes, can't concentrate etc. It symptoms include:

i. Irregular period or period might stop.

ii. Hot flashes

iii. Dryness of the vagina.

iv. Low libido

v. Difficult in getting pregnant.

21

7. Interstitial Cystitis (IC): this type of female reproductive system disorder, affect the bladder which will probably make you to lose your sex urge (libido) and cause extreme pain and problem peeing but can still conceive.

However, the possible symptoms for women suffering from this type of disorder include:

i. Stomach pain (in the lower abdomen)

ii. Frequent urge to pee.

iii. Frequent urination.

8. Abnormal uterine bleeding: this is the type of female reproductive system disorder where the woman will suffer from heavy or abnormal blood bleeding from the uterus abnormally or occurs at an irregular time, or after sex or between periods or for a longer period during menstruation or after menopause.

The possible causes of abnormal uterine bleeding are: Fibroids, uterine cancer and cervical cancer, PCOS, hormonal changes, uterine polyps, polycystic ovary syndrome, excess weight gain or loss, cervix or uterus infection, platelet dysfunction, anticoagulation and early pregnancy.

However, it possible symptoms include:

i.   Irregular or prolong period.

ii.   Heavy blood flow during menstruation (menorrhagia).

iii.   Bleeding during and after sex.

iv.   Heavy bleeding in-between period

What Are the Causes Or Sources Of Female Reproductive System Disorder?

Although, medically, each of the female reproductive system disorder have a cause or risk factor that can increase the chance of one suffering from it but my mentor (late Dr. Sebi) disagree with all that because to him, 'there is only one disease known as the compromising of the mucous membrane' that is, wherever the mucous membrane get broken or compromise, determine the type of disease that the patient might suffer from. That is, if the mucous membrane get broken or compromise in the lungs, the patient can suffer from COPD, pneumonia, cystic fibrosis etc., if it is compromised in the pancreas,

23

'diabetes', if it's in the trachea, the patient might suffer from wheezing, stridor or hemoptysis. If it is in the reproductive system, the patient might suffer from fibroid, endometriosis, infertility, PCOS etc.

In summary, the source of any type or form of female reproductive system disorder, is the compromising of the mucous membrane at the female reproductive system or any of its organs and the only way to get rid of the root-cause is through an intra-cellular cleansing which has to do with the cleansing of each cells of the body as the entire body system is connected to each other. So, if you cleanse some cells without cleansing the others, the other cells will be contaminated by the un-cleans cells. To do this, you will need to cleanse the following:

1. Colon
2. Lymph glands
3. Liver
4. Gallbladder
5. Kidney and the Skin.

CHAPTER TWO
Natural Cure for Female Reproductive System Disorders
How To Treat and Prevent Female Reproductive System Disorder?

Most of the female reproductive system disorder can be treated medically through surgery, medications and intrauterine insemination. However, according to late Dr. Sebi, all these options above are very expensive an ineffective with a very severe side effect and that the only way to treat and prevent any form or types of female reproductive system disorder is to reverse the body system to its original alkaline state where it's impossible for disease to survive. The question I know you will be asking yourself is 'How do I reverse my body system to its original alkaline state?' Dr. Sebi states that, you can reverse your entire body system back to its original alkaline state through the 2 steps of healings known as:

1. Cleansing of the entire body system through an intra-cellular cleansing. This means that each cells of the body will be rid of mucus (toxin) thereby making the body to be free from disease.

25

2. Revitalizing of the body system to recover, replenish and nourished the entire body to recover from all the energy that it must have lost as a result of the disease that the body must have suffered from.

3. The last thing to look at is to go back to nature and eat foods that are in Dr. Sebi nutritional guide (alkaline diets).

Please note that, the last thing is not part of Dr. Sebi two steps of healing but it's very important for the first two to work perfectly.

What Are the Types Of Cleansing And the Best One for Female Reproductive System Disorder?

Although there are various types of cleansing that people all over the world are aware of but I will only talk about the one recommended by late Dr. Sebi 'fasting'.

However, the types of fasting under cleansing are:

1. **Dry fasting:** just like the names, you will not eat anything completely except for the cleansing herbs.

2. **Liquid fasting**: under this type of fasting, you will

consume only liquid content together with the cleansing herbal teas and spring water without taking alcohol. Please note that, juice, with fiber (smoothies) is not liquid.

3. **Water fasting:** this is the best form of cleansing as you will have the opportunity to drink lots of spring water which is very good for cleansing of the body. Furthermore, this type of cleansing allows you to drink lots of spring water and the cleansing herbs and abstain from consuming even juice and smoothies and anything that is solid.

4. **Fruit fasting:** under this type of fasting, you consume only fruits that are in late Dr. Sebi nutritional guide, including smoothie that is made with fruit and the cleansing herbs. This is the second important type of fasting as people with some health challenges that can't do the water fast, can go for this type of fasting. The truth is, when I am doing fruit fasting, I consume smoothies and veggies which makes me to call it, smoothie and raw veggie fast.

5. **Smoothie fasting:** as earlier said, I named my fruits fasting 'smoothie and raw veggie fast' because, fruits are what you need to make smoothies and sometimes, we don't look at fruits as food that can satisfy us but believe smoothie can. Take your cleansing herbs and a gallon of spring water daily.

6. **Raw food fasting**: under this type of fasting, you are to eat only raw foods together with the cleansing herbs and at least a gallon of spring water daily.

Please note that, you will need to consume 1 gallon of spring water daily under each of the fasting that you decide to observe. Aside the cleansing herbs, you will also need to consume herbal tea made with Irish Sea moss and tamarind juice.

What Are The Possible Symptoms to Experience During Cleansing?

Because cleansing is an alternative medications that can be used to get rid of the root-cause of any type of disease, there are some symptoms that might sprang up while undergoing cleansing. These symptoms are:

1. Difficult to sleep or wakefulness

2. Discoloration of the tongue

3. Might be experiencing cold and flu

4. Might experience ache, pain, rashes and sometimes itching.

5. Experience some abnormal bowel movement

6. Experience fatigue (low energy)

7. Low blood pressure. Although this symptoms is very rare

8. Break outs and mucus will be expelled from the body.

How Long Do I Need to Get Rid of the Root-cause of Female Reproductive System Disorder?

The durations needed to rid of your body system of the root-cause of female reproductive system depends on your body's toxicity and level of tolerance.

According to Dr. Sebi, he cleanse (water fast) for 90 days when he was diagnose of impotence, diabetes and other disease and he recommends that, 1-3 month is the ideal duration for cleanse but 7-14 days is still workable.

29

However, people suffering from one health disorder or the other who cannot fast on water, can fast on fruit and raw veggies from late Dr. Sebi's nutritional guide. Don't be disturbed as both the water and smoothies and raw veggies fast will provide same result, the only difference is the time to get the result. So, I encourage 30days fast for people fasting on smoothies and raw veggies and 14days for water fast.

CHAPTER THREE
Goodbye to Female Reproductive System Disorders
What Are the Steps to Get Rid of the Root-cause of Female Reproductive System Disorder?

The steps to get rid of the root-cause of female reproductive system disorder are:

1. Stick to Dr. Sebi nutritional guide (alkaline diets) 100%

2. Observe water fast for 14 days or smoothie and raw veggie fast for 30days.

3. During the fasting period, consume at least a gallon of spring water daily, herbal cleansing teas and tamarind juice throughout the fasting (cleansing period).

4. Engage in routine exercise.

5. Immediately after the cleansing (fasting) period, take the herbal revitalizing teas for 14 days.

6. Observes the Does and don'ts of late Dr. Sebi

What Are Dr. Sebi Nutritional Guide?

Dr. Sebi nutritional guide is also known as 'Dr. Sebi Diet'. It is an African Bio-mineral balances (strictly alkaline) that the doctor put together to help reverse the body system to its original alkaline state. According to the late doctor, people fall sick because of the compromising of the mucous membrane which is as a result of the acidic or non-alkaline diet that we have filled our body system with that has made the body vulnerable to disease. However, in other to prevent any future diseases after the 2 steps of healing, we will need to retrace our steps back to nature and eat only alkaline diets thereby boosting our immune system, strengthening and repairing of our cells and making our body a disease-free zone. The various foods to eat are listed below:

The List of Fruits:

1. Apples
2. Avocado
3. Bananas (smallest and burros)
4. Berries
5. Cantaloupe

6. Cherries

7. Chirimoya sugar apple

8. Coconuts (soft jelly)

9. Cucumber

10. Currants

11. Dates

12. Elderberries

13. Figs

14. Grapes (seeded)

15. key limes (seeded)

16. Mangoes

17. Melon (seeded)

18. Orange Seville or sour

19. Papayas

20. peaches

21. pears

22. plums

23. prickly pears

24. Prunes

25. Raisins (seeded)

26. soursop

27.tamarind

The List of Vegetables:

1. Amaranth Greens

2. Asparagus

3. Bell peppers

4. Cactus flower

5. Chickpeas

6. Dandelion greens

7. Kale

8. Lettuce (excluding iceberg)

9. Mexican Cactus (Nopales)

10.Mexican Squash (Chayote)

11.Mushrooms (excluding shiitake)

12.Okra

13.Olives

14.Onions

15.Sea vegetables

16.Squash

17.Tomatoes (cherry and plum)

18.Wild Arugula

19.Zucchini

The List of Grains:

1. Amaranth
2. Fonio
3. Kamut
4. Khorasan wheat (kamut)
5. Quinoa
6. Rye
7. Spelt
8. Teff
9. Wild rice

The Lists of Flour:

i. Quinoa flour
ii. Rye flour
iii. Spelt flour
iv. Teff flour

The List of Nuts and Seeds:

1. Brazil nuts
2. Garbanzo Beans (chickpeas)
3. Hazelnut

4. Hemp seeds

5. Sesame seeds (raw)

6. Tahini butter (raw)

7. Walnuts

The List of Oils:

1. Avocado oil

2. Coconut oil (uncooked)

3. Grape seed oil

4. Hempseed oil

5. Olive oil (uncooked),

6. Sesame oil

The List of Spices:

1. Achiote

2. Agave syrup (pure)

3. Basil

4. Bay leaf

5. Cayenne

6. Cloves dill

7. Date sugar

8. Granulated seaweed (powdered)

9. Habanero

10. Oregano

11. Onion powder

12. Sage

13. Sea salt (pure)

14. Sweet basil

15. Tarragon

16. Thyme

How Do I Observe My Fast (Cleansing)?

I won't bug you with stringent and cumbersome steps by step process to fast deciding what you do from the first hour of your fast to the last. But will get you through a simplified way to make it flexible for you to be able to undergo the fast without any difficulty.

Did I say without any difficulty? That is not true because there is no way you are going to fast for 14day (water fast) or 30day (smoothies and raw veggie fast) that you will say it's not difficult. The good news is; you are paying the price for that baby that you have long desire to hold tight on your hands and live a healthy life.

However, to observe your fast, start your day (everyday) with a cup of herbal tea made with Irish Sea moss and another cup of tamarind juice.

Before leaving the house for work, engage in some light exercise such as walking or skipping or bicycle riding etc.

After every two hours, take a cup or two of spring water irrespective of the type of fast you are observing.

From 8-10am, any time that is convenient for you; take a cup of herbal cleansing tea made with prodigiosa leaves, eucalyptus and elderberries and another cup of tea made with cascara sagrada, Rhubard root and dandelion leaves.

That should be all in the morning if you are observing water fast but if you are on smoothie and raw veggie fast, you can make a delicious smoothie for breakfast.

By noon, within the range of 12-2pm, which ever time is convenient for you; take the herbal cleansing tea made with prodigiosa leaves, eucalyptus and elderberries and another cup of tea made with cascara sagrada, Rhubard root and dandelion leaves.

Please note that, the consumption of 1 gallon of spring water per day is very important so, look at a suitable time to consume at least a cup or two after every 2hours. You can as well drink more than a gallon but you are not to consume less than a gallon per day during your cleansing period.

For the smoothie and raw veggie fasters, you can snacks on some of the fruits that are in late Dr. Sebi nutritional guide.

In the evening within the range of 4-6pm, take the herbal cleansing tea made with prodigiosa leaves, eucalyptus and elderberries and another cup of tea made with cascara sagrada, Rhubard root and dandelion leaves.

For smoothie and raw veggie fasters, you can prepare vegetable or fruits salad as dinner. Ensure you have a journal that you tag as "My Fasting/Cleanse Journal" to record your daily experience.

How Do I Take the Herbal Cleansing Teas to Get Rid of the Root-cause of Female Reproductive System Disorder?

Instead of taking a bout 5-6 cups of herbs, I combine 2-3 herbs to make a single tea to prevent you from consuming lots of water which might prevent you from consuming the required amount of spring water per day. However, to maintain the concentration, I make sure you don't combine more than 3herbs together. Follow the steps below for a simplified way to mix the herbs together:

1. In the morning from 6-8am, take a cup of herbal tea made with Irish Sea Moss. Within that same range of time, take a cup of tamarind juice ensure you consume a cup or two of spring water after every 2hours.

2. By 8-10am, 12-2pm and 4-6pm, take a cup of herbal cleansing tea made with prodigiosa leaves, eucalyptus and elderberries for 14days if you are on water fast and 30days if you are on smoothie and raw veggie fast.

3. Within this same time. That is, 8-10am, 12-2pm and 4-6pm, take a cup of herbal cleansing tea made with cascara sagrada, Rhubard root and ½ tablespoon of Dandelion infusion for 14days if you are on water fast and 30days if you are on smoothie and raw veggie fast.

Please note that, you have to be drinking a cup or two of spring water after every 2hours to enable you meets the targeted amount of spring water (1gallon) per day.

How Do I Prepare Herbal Tea With Irish Sea Moss?

To prepare herbal tea with Irish Sea moss, you will have to take the following steps:

1. Measure 8-10ounce of water and boil the water in your ceramic pot or saucepan.
2. Once the water is boiled, drop it down and measure 2-3 tablespoon of Irish Sea moss (powder form) or 1teaspoon (liquid form) and add it to the boiled water.

41

3. Cover the mixture for about 10-15 minutes to dissolve all the dissolvable and use your strainer to strain it.

4. For the dosage, take a cup of Irish Sea moss once per day throughout the period of your cleansing and revitalization.

How Do I Prepare Tamarind Juice?

To prepare tamarind juice, take the steps below:

1. Get a cup of tamarind pods and peel it or a block of tamarind.

2. Measure 16-20ounce of water and boil it.

3. Pour the boiled water into the tamarind pods or the block and leave it for 10hours or overnight.

4. Use a strainer to strain it into glass pitcher and store it in the refrigerator.

5. Drink 8ounce daily for the period of your cleanse.

How Do I Prepare Herbal Cleansing Tea with Prodigiosa Leaves, Eucalyptus Leaves and Elderberries?

To prepare herbal cleansing tea with prodigiosa leaves, eucalyptus leaves and elderberries, take the steps below:

1. First, you will have to make sure all the herbs are ready. To avoid too much stress, you can order each herb online and you will get it dried, chopped and well packaged. Alternatively, you can get all the herbs in a nursery garden, wash and dry each herb separately until they are dried before chopping or pounding the herbs separately.

2. Measuring 10-12ounce of water and add (pour) it to your saucepan and boil it.

3. Once the water is boiling, measure 1tablespoon of dried elderberries and pours it into the boiling water.

4. Reduce the hotness of your fire (gas) and allow the mixture to boil for at least 15 minutes.

5. Step it down and measure 1 teaspoon each of prodigiosa and eucalyptus dried leaves and add it to

the boil mixture with elderberries.

6. Cover it for 15-minutes and strain it into your tea cup/mug.

7. You are done. Take 3 cups (10ounce) daily.

How Do I Prepare Herbal Cleansing Tea with Cascara Sagrada, Rhubard Root and Dandelion?

In other to make herbal cleansing tea with these three herbs, take the steps below:

1. First and foremost, you will need to have all the herbs at hand. Order the herbs online or harvest them by getting the bark of cascara sagrada, Rhubard root and dandelion leaves. Please note that, FRESH LEAVES OF DANDALION IS THE BEST.

2. Wash the fresh leaves of dandelion to remove all the dirt on it.

3. After washing the dandelion leaves, measure ½-1 cup of the washed dandelion and add (pour) it into

your saucepan or pot.

4. Measure 40-50ounce of water and boil it. Once the water is boiled, turn it into your saucepan or pot where the dandelion leaves are and cover the mixture for at least 12 hours or overnight (throughout the night) for it to be completely infused.

5. After the twelve hours or the next day, get a strainer and strain it into a cup.

6. Measure 8ounce of water and 1 teaspoon of the cascara sagrada bark and the Rhubard root and boil the mixture for 15-20 minutes.

7. Step it down and strain it using a strainer into your tea cup/mug.

8. Measure ½ tablespoon of Dandelion infusion and add it to the strain cascara sagrada bark and Rhubard root's tea and stir it. You are done!

How Do I Take My Revitalizing Herbs?

The cleansing herbs are design to cleanse your body system whereas the revitalizing herbs are to get rid of the female reproductive system disorder completely, replenish and nourish the body system and restore it to its original alkaline state. However, the ways to take these herbal teas are as follows:

1. If you finish cleansing today (either on the 14th day for water fast or 30days for smoothie and raw veggie fast), by the next day (15th for water fast and 31st for smoothie and raw veggie fast) you should start consuming your revitalizing herbs.

2. By 6-8am, take a cup of herbal tea made with Irish Sea moss for the 14days of your revitalizing period.

3. Use the ¼ of the Pau D'Arco infusion (will talk about how to make the infusion soon) to flush your vagina every morning for the 14 days of your revitalization.

4. Within the range of 8-10 am, you will take 3cups of herbal revitalizing tea. One made with Pau D'Arco. Another cup made with Red raspberries leaves,

shepherd purse and red cloves and the last cup with stinging nettle and peony.

5. Within the range of time from 12-2pm, whenever it's convenient for you, repeat the same 3 cups of herbal revitalizing teas.

6. By 4-6pm, repeat the same revitalizing herbal teas.

7. Remember that during revitalizing, you are not fasting so you can eat whatever you want to just make sure to consume the revitalizing herbs but I strongly advise that you eat only foods that are in late Dr. Sebi nutritional guide or alkaline diets.

Please note that, it's the same way that we prepare Irish Sea moss during cleansing that you will use to prepare it again during revitalizing.

How Do I Prepare Herbal Revitalizing Tea with Pau D'Arco?

To prepare herbal revitalizing tea with Pau D'Arco, take the steps below:

1. Harvest the bark of Pau D'Arco, dry it and chop it

into smaller pieces or you can place an order online and it will come chopped, dried and package.

2. Measure 32-40ounce of water and 4 teaspoon of the bark of Pau D'Arco into the water and boil the mixture for 15-20 minutes.

3. Step it down and allow it to get cold.

4. Use a strainer to strain it into a glass pitcher Put off the fire and allow it to get cold for at least 30minutes to an hour.

5. You should use filter or strainer to strain the bark from the water.

6. Share it into 4 places and use ¼ to flush your vagina every morning and take the remaining ¾ morning afternoon and evening everyday throughout your revitalizing days.

How Do I Prepare Herbal Revitalizing Tea with Red Raspberries Leaves, Shepherd Purse and Red Clovers?

To prepare herbal revitalizing tea with Red raspberries leaves, shepherd purse and red clovers, you will need to take the steps below:

1. Get all the three herbs available. You can order it online and they will come dried, chopped and packaged separately.
2. Boil 8-10 ounce of water.
3. Measure 1teaspoon each of red clovers and shepherd's purse extract and 1½teaspoon of raspberries leaves and pour it into your tea cup/mug.
4. Pour the boiled water into your tea cup or mug with the herbs and cover it for 15-20minutes.
5. You are good. Take these herbal teas 3cups (8-10) daily throughout the 14days of your revitalizing process.

How Do I Prepare Herbal Revitalizing Tea with Stinging Nettle and Peony Extract?

To make herbal revitalizing tea with stinging nettle and peony, you will have to take the steps below:

1. Get all the two herbs available or you can place an order online and the herbs will come chopped, dried and packaged.

2. Measure 8-10ounce of water and boil it.

3. Measure 1teaspoon of stinging nettle extract and pour it into your tea cup and pour the boil water into the tea cup.

4. Cover it for 8-10 minutes before measuring 2 teaspoon of peony extract and pour it inside the tea cup with the stinging nettle and cover it for additional 5-7minutes.

5. You are done. Take a cup (8ounce) of this herbal revitalizing tea 3days daily for the 14 days of your revitalizing process.

What Are the Does and Don'ts to Eliminate the Root-cause of Female Reproductive System Disorders?

Not just about the female reproductive system disorder, but to live a healthy and sick free life, there are some does and don'ts that one must abide by. They include:

1. Eat only foods that are in late Dr. Sebi nutritional guide (alkaline diet) because if you keep eating acidic food, your entire body system will be vulnerable to disease again. Irrespective of the disease that you just treat yourself of, if you continue eating acidic food, you might suffer from same disease again.

2. Ensure you undergo cleansing of the body (intra-cellular) for a period of 7day at least once a year if you stick to eating only alkaline diet (Dr. Sebi nutritional guide) but if you still go back eating anything eatable that is acidic and non-alkaline diet, then you will need to undergo the cleansing process for at least 7days after every three month.

3. Drink at least a gallon of spring water daily.

4. Endure you don't eat anything that is microwaves.

5. Eat foods that can help to repairs, strengthen and rebuild your cells and boost your immune system.

6. Do not consume sugary and starchy food as they have the potency to cause inflammation and outbreak.

7. Ensure you use water fast to undergo the cleansing process except if you have some health conditions that you can opt in for smoothie and raw veggie fast.

8. Once you are done with cleansing, begging the revitalization process. That is, if you finish cleansing today, by tomorrow, you can start with the revitalizing process.

CHAPTER FOUR
Review of the Cleansing Herbs
What Are the Cleansing Herbs to Get Rid of the Root-cause of Female Reproductive System Disorders?

The cleansing herbs to get rid of female reproductive system disorders are:

1. Irish Sea Moss

2. Prodigiosa

3. Eucalyptus

4. Elderberries

5. Cascara sagrada

6. Rhubard root

7. Dandelion

What Is Sea Moss?

Irish Sea moss is one of the best electrical herbs that late Dr. Sebi recommended for both the cleansing and revitalizing of the body system to get rid of the root-cause of female reproductive system disorder. This herb belongs to the family of red algae species and it's loaded with lots of nutrient, mineral and vitamins. In fact, these herbs contain over 92 out of the 102 minerals that the body needs to stay healthy.

However, consuming of herbal teas made with Irish Sea moss helps to boost, calm and heal the immune and thyroid system, repairs and strengthen cells, calm and relief digestion and respiratory tract disorder, serves as anti-aging (prevents skin wrinkling), get rid of joints pains, joints swelling, arthritis and other pain caused by inflammation, enrich mood, boost energy and eradicate fatigue, anxieties and fussiness, fight against cold, flu and various infections disease and skin disorder like; acne, skin inflammation disease etc.

Till at the time of publishing this book, Irish sea moss' herbal teas is safe for consumption except if used in large quantity (abused) that one might experience some mild side effect like:

1. Itching throat or burning sensation on the mouth and sometimes the throat.
i. Throwing up or nausea
ii. Stomach upset or irritation

iii. Sometimes, one might experience fever

Please note that, all these side effects only happen when you abuse the herbs.

What Are the Not-full Precautions before Consuming of Irish Sea Moss' Tea?

Irish Sea moss is loaded with iron which is the major factor that can trigger hypothyroidism; therefore, any person suffering from hypothyroidism should not use this herb without consulting with their health administrator or doctor.

Does Irish Sea Moss' Tea Interact With Any Medications?

Yes. Teas made with Irish Sea moss interacts with all types of medications made for thyroid disorders. For clarity sake, if you are suffering from any type of thyroid disorder, consult your health administrator or doctor first before consuming Irish Sea moss' tea.

Please note that the dosage and how to prepare it have

been talked about in the last chapter.

What Is Prodigiosa?

Prodigiosa is another interesting perennial plant from daisy family that is always covered with a bushy large leaves and flowers. Late Dr. Sebi recommended this herb as part of the herbs for the cleansing of the body system to get rid of female reproductive system disorder because of how effective the herb is and how the herbs have been in used for over centuries for the treatment and prevention of various health disorder such as; diabetes, stomach irritation, diarrhea, arthritis, aching joints, gallbladder disease, improve digestion of fat by synthesis of bile in the liver and treat chronic gastritis, cataracts and lots more.

One amazing fact about this herb is that, it does not have any side effect to be worried about.

What Are the Note-Full Precautions before Consuming of Prodigiosa's Tea?

The   note-full   precautions   before   consuming   of

Prodigiosa's tea are:

i. It is very important for nursing mothers and pregnant women to know much about what they consume. However, since there is little to say about the effect of these herbs on nursing and pregnant women, I advise that they stay off this herb.

ii. People suffering from type 1 diabetes should not consume Prodigiosa's tea and people with type 2 diabetes should make sure they control their sugar level if they want to consume this tea.

iii. Do not consume Prodigiosa's tea two weeks before and after surgery because it controls blood sugar level.

Does Prodigiosa's Tea Interact with Any Medications?

Yes. Because of how effective the tea made with prodigiosa leaves is in lowering of blood sugar level, consuming Prodigiosa's tea with any type of diabetes medication will lead to over lowering of blood sugar level.

What Is Eucalyptus Tree?

Eucalyptus tree is another amazing herb that is from the native of Australia and both the leaves and the bark of this plant have been used for over a century in Australia and for thousands of years by the Greek, Chinese, and Indian Ayurvedic people for the treatment of various health disorders. However, late Dr. Sebi recommended this herb for the cleansing of the body system for female reproductive system disorder because tea made from the leaves of this plant is a very effective plant-based anti-oxidants that has the potency to relief and treat bronchitis, diabetes, pains and swollen that is caused by inflammation, cleanse and purify the skin, reduce inflammation, serves an anti-fungi, anti-bacteria and anti-viral that fight against the activities of harmful microorganism, control blood sugar level, sooth joint and muscle pain, build and repair damage muscle, treat and prevent cold, cough, congestion, sore throat, sinusitis asthma, dental plaque, gallbladder, liver and bladder disease, skin disease, ulcer etc.

Tea made with the leaves of eucalyptus is 100% safe for everybody to consume including children, pregnant and

58

breast-feeding mothers but eucalyptus oil is not safe as applying it oil directly to the skin without being diluted can lead to severe nervous system disorder.

What Are the Note-Full Precautions before Consuming of Eucalyptus' Tea?

There is nothing to be worried about in regards the tea made with Eucalyptus leaves but the oil is not safe as it can cause seizure or even death when used on infant/children.

Do not consume eucalyptus tea two weeks before and after surgery because it has the potency to lower blood sugar level.

Does Eucalyptus' Tea Interact with Any Medications?

Yes. Eucalyptus' teas interact with all diabetes medications as both the tea and the medications have the same potency to lower blood sugar level. Therefore, consuming both the tea and diabetes medication can lead to over lowering of blood sugar level.

What Is Elderberry?

Elderberry is a flowering plant belonging to the Adoxaceae's family that both the fruits (berries) and the leaves have been used for more than centuries for the treatment and prevention of various health disorders. However, Dr. Sebi recommended this herb for the cleansing of the body system for female reproductive system disorder because of how effective the tea serves as an immune booster, natural laxative, diuretic, anti-inflammatory, anti-bacterial, anti-oxidants and how effective it cleanse and detox the entire body system by inducing urine production and sweat and eliminate mucus from the upper respiratory system and the lungs and reduce damages that are caused by oxidative stress. However, tea made with this herb is very effective for the treatment of different types of infectious diseases such as; sciatica, influenza etc., it also helps to relief and treat pain and swollen that is caused by inflammation, treat and prevent various health disorders such as: constipation, skin disorder, chronic fatigue syndrome, depression, anxiety, flu and cold, nerve and heart disorder, various types of cancer etc.

The most amazing thing about this herb is the fact that it's 100% safe for consumption but since elderberry contains some compound, I recommend you don't consume this herb for more than 12weeks but if you must, take a break for a week or two before you can start taking it again.

What Are the Notable Precaution before Consuming Elderberry's Tea?

The notable precautions before consuming of elderberry's tea are as follows:

i. Since there is little or no information as to the effect of these herbs on nursing and breast-feeding mothers, I advise that, they should not consume this herb.

ii. Children should not consume these herbs and teenagers should not consume it for more than 14days at stretch.

iii. Since tea made with elderberries have the potency to boost the immune system, people suffering from any form of auto-immune disease such as; multiple sclerosis, rheumatoid arthritis, lupus etc. should not use this herb without their doctor's approval.

Does Elderberry's Tea Interact with Any Medications?

Yes. Any medication made to boost or decrease the functions of immune system will interact with elderberry's tea as it will either increase or decrease the effect of the medication.

What Is Cascara Sagrada?

Cascara sagrada is another amazing shrub plant that belongs to the Rhamnaceae's family. Although this herb is no longer sold as over the counter drugs after FDA declares in 2002 that the plant does not meet the requirement to be sold as over the counter drugs (OTC). Irrespective of what FDA declare, my mentor, late Dr. Sebi still add this herb as part of the cleansing herb for female reproductive system disorder because of its effectiveness in serving as a purgative for constipation and laxation and how effective it is in cleansing (detoxifying) of the colon. Furthermore, this herb is very effective for the treatment and prevention of various health challenges such as: joint and muscle pain, gallstones, various types of cancer, liver and digestive disorder, dysentery, sexually transmitted disease such as; gonorrhea, herpes etc. in addition, tea made with cascara sagrada's bark is save if consume for a week but if consume for more than a week constantly, there are chances of some possible side effects. The possible side effects to experience are:

i. Stomach cramps or upset
ii. Heart disorder (rare)
iii. Drying up
iv. Weakness of the muscle weakness (rare)

What Are the Note-full Precautions before Consuming of Cascara Sagrada's Tea?

The note-full precautions before consuming of Cascara Sagrada's tea are as follows:

i. Cascara Sagrada has the potency to induce labor. So, pregnant women should not consume Cascara

Sagrada's tea as it can cause miscarriage and nursing mothers should not consume this tea as it might make the infant to suffer from diarrhea.

ii. Cascara sagrada's tea should not be given to children as they will get dehydrated thereby losing electrolytes like potassium.

iii. If you are suffering from stomach upset without any reasonable cause, ulcerative colitis or Crohn's disease, intestinal obstruction, kidney disorder, hemorrhoids do not consume cascara sagrada's tea.

Does Cascara Sagrada's Tea Interact with Any Medications?

Yes. Cascara Sagrada's tea interacts with the under-listed medications:

1. All inflammation medications: all inflammation medications are design to reduce potassium in the body and Cascara Sagrada has the same potency. Therefore, combining both Cascara Sagrada's tea with any medications for inflammation will over lower the level of potassium in the body thereby

leading to dehydration and potassium deficiency.

2. All Stimulant laxatives: Cascara Sagrada has the potency to lower potassium in the body just like any stimulant laxative. So, consuming cascara sagrada with any stimulant laxative like 'Digoxin (lanoxin)' will lead to potassium deficiency in the body.

What Is Rhubarb Root?

Rhubarb Root is the root of Rhubarb plant that Dr. Sebi recommended its tea as an effective cleansing herb for female reproductive system disorders. Tea made from this plant has been in used for more than century by the Chinese as a natural laxative to treat and prevent health disorders such as: diarrhea, pains caused by inflammation, pancreatitis, cold and canker sores, gastrointestinal (GI) bleeding, digestive disorder, enhance digestive tract health and purifies the blood by eliminating of heavy metal from the bloodstream, relief dysmenorrhea (menstrual cramp), fight against harmful microorganism such as herpes simplex virus, shed excess body weight (cholesterol), improve menopausal symptoms and respiratory system of people suffering from ARDS to enjoy a better and healthier breath, prevent and stop stomach bleeding and lots more!

There is nothing to worry about as Rhubard root's tea is 100% safe for consumption but tea made with the leaves is not safe because it contains oxalic acid that can cause some possible side effect.

What Are the Note-full Precautions before Consuming Rhubarb Root's Tea?

The note-full precautions before consuming of Rhubard root's tea are as follows:

i.   Since there are no much information to ascertain the effect of Rhubard root's tea on nursing mothers and pregnant women, I advise that they don't consume these herbs.

ii. People suffering from kidney stone or kidney and liver disorder should not consume Rhubarb root's tea as it can worsen their situation.

Does Rhubard Root's Tea Interact with Any Medications?

Yes. Rhubard root's tea interact medications such as:

1. All medication for inflammation: all medications for inflammation lower potassium in the body. So, consuming both Rhubard root's tea and medication for inflammation will lead to dehydration and potassium deficiency.

2. All laxatives medications: consuming both Rhubard root's tea with laxatives will lead to potassium deficiency.

3. Medication that can harm the kidney: since Rhubard root's tea has potency to harm the kidney, consuming of this herb and any medications that have same potency will increase the risk of kidney problem.

What Is Dandelion?

Dandelion is one of the best plants that Dr. Sebi included as parts of the cleansing herbs for people suffering from female reproductive system disorders. This plant have been in used all over the world for more than a century for the treatment of various health challenges such as: swelling (inflammation) of the pancreas, tonsils (tonsillitis), bladder or urethra disorder, digestive disorders, boost the immune system to fight against disease and various infections, cleansing of the kidney, gallbladder, purifies blood, blood stream and the entire body system by inducing urine production, treat and prevent cancer by destroying cancer cells and preventing it from mutating, inhibit crystals from forming in the urine, treat kidney and liver disorders, diabetes by regulating blood sugar level in the body, high blood pressure by eliminating of excess fluid in the body, urinary disorder, combat inflammation and relief pains that are cause by inflammation, it neutralize the negative effects of free radicals in the body, shed excess body weight by promoting carbohydrate metabolism and lots more.

Dandelion infusion is completely safe for consumption but if abused, one might suffer from some mild side effects like:

1. Stomach irritation

2. Diarrhea

i. Heartburn (very rare)

ii. Allergic reactions

What Are the Not-full Precautions before Consuming of Dandelion's Infusion?

The note-full precautions before consuming of dandelion's infusion are:

i. Since there is little or no information in respect to the negative effects of dandelion on pregnant and nursing mothers, I strongly advise that they stay of the consumption of this infusion.

ii. People suffering from blood bleeding of any form, eczema or allergic to plant from the marigold or ragweed family, please do not consume dandelion's infusion as it has the potency to slow down blood clotting thereby increasing the chance of bleeding and bruising and causes eczema reaction.

iii. People suffering from kidney failure, should not consume dandelion's infusion.

Does Dandelion's Infusion Interact with Any Medications?

Yes. Dandelion's infusion does interact with some medications such as:

1. All antibiotics medications.
2. Medications that have diuretic effect
3. All medications changed by the liver.

CHAPTER FIVE
Review of the Revitalizing Herbs
What Are the Revitalizing Herbs to Get Rid of the Root-cause of Female Reproductive System Disorders?

The revitalizing herbs to get rid of the root-cause of female reproductive system disorders are:

1. Irish Sea Moss (I have written about this herb under the cleansing herbs)
2. Pau D'Arco
3. Red Raspberries
4. Shepard's purse
5. Red clovers
6. Stinging nettle
7. Peony

What Is Pau D'Arco?

Pau D'Arco is an amazing herbal plant (tree) that is common in tropical rainforests. Late Dr. Sebi include this herb as part of the revitalizing herb to get rid of the root-cause of female reproductive system disorders because of its potency to cleanse the body and fight against various infection caused by; bacteria, viruses and fungi. Such infection are; methicillin-resistant Staphylococcus aureus (MRSA), pylori, herpes simplex virus I and II, poliovirus, vesicular stomatitis virus, Helicobacter (H.) influenza etc. the bark of this tree is also used for the treatment of some health challenges such as: candida, cancer, ulcer, relief and reduce pain caused by inflammation, cancer and arthritis etc.

Furthermore, this herb is safe for consumption but if abused, it can lead to some mild side effect like:

1. Giddiness
2. Diarrhea
3. Unsettled stomach
4. Queasiness

What Are the Note-full Precautions before Consuming of Pau D'Arco's Infusion?

The note-full precautions before consuming of Pau D'Arco's Infusion are:

1. Do not consume the Pau D'Arco's infusion 2 weeks before and after surgery as it will increase the risk of bleeding.

2. Since there is little or no information as to the negative effect of Pau D'Arco's infusion on nursing mothers and pregnant women, I advise they don't consume Pau D'Arco's infusion.

Does Pau D'Arco's Infusion Interact with Any Medications?

Yes. Pau D'Arco's infusion interacts with all medications design to slow blood clotting.

What Is Red Raspberry Leaves?

Red raspberry leaves are the leaves of the plant that produces red raspberry. This plant is an amazing herbal plant as both the fruit and leaves are used for medicinal purpose for many centuries ago. However, this herb was added by Dr. Sebi for the revitalization of the body after cleansing for female reproductive system disorder because of its potency to ease the pain of labor and delivery, treat gastrointestinal (GI) disorders such as; gargle, diarrhea, sore throat, cold and flu, skin disorder such as; rashes and eczema. It also helps to treat and prevent abnormal uterine bleeding, heavy blood flow during menstruation (period), dysmenorrhea (menstrual cramp), boost the heart's health and prevent heart's failure or disorders, lower and control blood sugar level (diabetes), lower blood pressure and prevent infant miscarriage etc.

This herb is 100% safe for consumption with no single trace of side effect.

What Are the Note-Full Precautions before Consuming Red Raspberry's Tea?

The note-full precautions before consuming of red raspberry's tea are:

1. Women that find it difficult to get pregnant or early pregnant women and nursing mothers should not consume red raspberry's tea as there is no much

information to determine the side effect of the tea on them.

2. People suffering with sugar issue such as diabetes should avoid the use of this herb but if they must consume it, they must make sure their blood sugar level is monitored.

3. People suffering from hormone-sensitive conditions should consult with their doctors before consuming of this herbal tea.

Does Red Raspberry's Tea Interact with Any Medications?

No. red raspberry's tea can be taken with any other medication with nothing to worry about.

What Is Shepherd's Purse?

Shepherd's purse is another interesting herb that belongs to the Cruciferae family. This herb was first used during WWI as an anti-blood bleeding remedy to stop the bleeding of blood in Britain in the absence of goldenseal and ergot. This herb was added as herbs for revitalizing of the body system after revitalizing of the body system for female reproductive system disorder because of its; astringent, diuretic and antiseptic properties which makes it effective in stimulating of circulation, staunching of mucous membrane bleeding and blood bleeding such as: hemorrhage, abnormal and heavy blood bleeding during menstruation (period), postpartum bleeding, uterine bleeding, nose bleeding and treat and prevent: gallbladder inflammation (cystitis), premenstrual syndrome (PMS), menorrhagia (menstrual cramp), calculosis, lower blood pressure, induce labor and childbirth (delivery), relief and treat headache, varicose veins and promote fast wound healings

However, tea made from this herb is 100% safe for consumption in less than a month but if it is abused for a long period of time, it can lead to some mild side effect like:

1. Heart tremors
2. Lethargy
3. Blood pressure swing
4. Thyroid malfunctioning

What Are the Note-full Precautions before Consuming of Shepherd's Purse Tea?

The note-full precautions before consuming of Shepherd's purse tea are:

1. Shepherd's purse tea is strictly for adult above the age of 17.
2. Since it can induce labor and cause miscarriage for pregnant women, they should not consume Shepherd's purse tea.
3. Since there is little or no information in respect to the negative effect of Shepherd's purse tea on nursing mothers, I advise that they don't consume Shepherd's purse tea.
4. People suffering from severe heart disorder, kidney stones (nephrolithiasis) and thyroid disorder should not consume Shepherd's purse tea.

Does Shepherd's Purse Tea Interact with Any Medications?

Yes. Shepherd's purse tea interacts with some certain medications. They include:

i. All medications for thyroid hormone: since Shepherd's purse tea regulate the production of thyroid hormone, consuming of thyroid hormone medications together with Shepherd's purse tea will render the medications ineffective.

ii. All sedative medications: Shepherd's purse tea is a natural laxative. So, consuming of the tea with any sedative medications will lead to excess sleepiness or too much sleep.

What Is Red Clover?

Red clover is a beautiful and good looking flowering plant that belongs to the Fabaceae's family and herbaceous species. The tops of red clover flower have been used for centuries for the treatment and prevention of various health challenges such as; hot flashes, premenstrual syndrome (PMS), sexually transmitted diseases (STDs) such as: herpes simplex virus and HIV, various types of cancer, mastalgia, hypercholesterolemia, skin sores, bronchitis, helps to develop female secondary sex characteristics, regulate menstrual cycle and a lots more. Apart from the above benefits, tea made with red clover also helps to purifies the blood by eliminating of heavy metal from the bloodstream, shrink fibroid tumors and relief its pain, treat and prevent endometriosis, mastalgia, bronchitis, vaginal discharge, promote bone density, strengthen vagina muscle and nervous system etc.

However, teas made with red clover are possibly safe for consumption but if abused, it can lead to some side effects which include:

i. Rash-like reactions

ii. Hemorrhage

iii. Headache

iv. Muscle aching.

v. Unsettled stomach

What Are the Note-full Precautions before Consuming Red Clover's Tea?

The note-full precautions before consuming red clover's tea are:

1. Pregnant and nursing mothers should not consume red clover's tea because it will lead to hormonal imbalances.

2. People suffering from blood bleeding disorders should not consume red clover's tea as it can increase the risk of bruising and bleeding.

3. Do not consume red clover's tea two weeks before and after surgery because of its potency to slow blood clotting.

4. People suffering from hormone-sensitive conditions such as; uterine, fibroids, ovarian and breast cancer should not consume red clover's tea.

Does Red Clover's Tea Interact with Any Medications?

Yes. Red clover's tea interacts with some certain medications like:

1. All types of birth control pills: since red clover's tea enhance the production of estrogen and all types of birth control have same potency, consuming both

red clovers' tea and any type of birth control pills will reduce the effect of birth control pills.

2. All types of estrogen pills: consuming of red clover's tea together with any estrogen pills will reduce the effect of the medications.

3. All medications that are change by the liver.

4. All types of medications that have the potency to slow blood clotting.

What Is Stinging Nettle?

Stinging nettle is a perennial and herbaceous flowering plant that belongs to the urticaceae's family that its root, stem and leaves have been used for medicinal purpose for over a century.

However, late Dr. Sebi adds this herb as a revitalizing herb after cleansing for female reproductive system disorder because it is very effective and powerful anti-oxidant, diuretic, anti-microbial, an astringent, anti-ulcer and pain-reliever that has the potency to reduce inflammation and ease pain that is caused by inflammation, treat and prevent health challenges such as: endocrine disorders, anemia, enlarged spleen, urinary tract infections (UTI), osteoarthritis, nephrolithiasis, stop internal and external blood bleeding such as; uterine bleeding, nosebleeds, bowel bleeding and other internal bleeding, enhance healthy circulation, decongest the lung, purifies the blood, helps with PMS and lots more.

Furthermore, this herb is safe for consumption for over two years at a stretch but if it is consume in overdose, you might suffer some mild side effect like:

1. Inflammations or rashes
2. Diarrhea
3. Stomach irritations
4. Sweltering
5. Urinary disorders

What Are the Note-full Precautions before Consuming of Stinging Nettle's Tea?

The note-full precautions before consuming of Stinging Nettle's Tea are:

1. Pregnant and nursing mothers should not consume Stinging Nettle's tea as it can cause miscarriage to pregnant women and for nursing mothers, much is not known about its negative effect.

2. People suffering from diabetes and high blood pressure should not consume Stinging Nettle's tea as it can over lower their blood sugar level and blood pressure respectively.

3. People suffering from kidney disorder should consult with their health administrator or doctor before consuming of Stinging Nettle's tea.

Does Stinging Nettle's Tea Interact with Any Type of Medications?

Yes. Stinging Nettle's tea interacts with some medications like:

1. All sedative medications: Since Stinging Nettle's tea is a natural sedative; consuming this tea with any sedative medications will lead to too much sleepiness.

2. All medications that slow blood clotting: Stinging Nettle's tea is loaded with vitamin K that helps to boost blood clotting. Consuming Stinging Nettle's tea with any medications with the potency to slow blood clotting will only reduce the effect of the medication.

3. All diabetes medications: since stinging nettle's tea has the potency to lower blood sugar level, consuming of Stinging Nettle's tea with any type of diabetes medication will lead to over lowering of blood sugar level.

What Is Peony?

Peony is a good-looking and beautiful flower that belongs to Paeonaceae's family. The flower of this plant is believed to be a protector from evil as some people believed that it helps to drive away evil from the house where it is placed at the door. At the same time it is used for the treatment of some health challenges. However, late Dr. Sebi include this herb as a revitalizing herbs after cleansing to get rid of the root-cause of female reproductive system disorder because of how potent it is as an anti-oxidant and astringent that is effective in the treatment and prevention of; menstrual cramps, premenstrual syndrome (PMS), polycystic ovary syndrome, hemorrhoids, chronic fatigue syndrome (CFS), viral hepatitis, spasms, migraine headaches, facial wrinkling, liver cirrhosis, muscle cramps, osteoarthritis, rheumatoid arthritis, stomach upset, convulsions, nervous disorder and nerve pain (neuralgia), prevent blood clotting, termination of early pregnancy, arteries hardening (atherosclerosis) etc.

Till at the time publishing this book, tea made with peony is 100% safe for consumption for a month but if abused and taken for more than a month, it can lead to these mild side effects:

i. Stomach irritation or cramp
ii. If it touches some sensitive part of your body, you might have rash.

What Are the Note-full Precautions before Consuming of Peony's Tea?

The note-full precautions before consuming of Peony's tea include:

i. Pregnant women should not consume Peony's tea because it can lead to miscarriage.

ii. There is no information to ascertain it negative effects on nursing mothers so I advise they shouldn't consume Peony's tea.

iii. Since it helps in slowing blood clotting, people with bleeding disorders shouldn't consume Peony's tea.

iv. Do not consume Peony's tea two weeks before and after surgery because it has the potency to slow down blood clotting and increase the risk of bleeding.

Does Peony's Tea Interact with Any Medications?

Yes. Peony's tea interacts with some certain medications like:

1. All medications that have the potency to slow down blood clotting: combining Peony's tea and medications that has the same potency will increase the risk of blood bleeding and bruising.

2. Children below the age of 17 should not consume this herb as it might lead to seizures.

About the Author

Clement Jacob is an African researcher, philanthropist, an herbalist and an astute student of late Dr. Sebi who studied and learns about how to use late Dr. Sebi 2 steps of healing methodology, alkaline herbs and diets to treat and prevent various health challenges.

According to the author, this book is a resource material to women that have lost hope of being a mother, who have experience countless miscarriage and have tried various pills and supplement to get pregnant but could not.

He further state that, this book is priceless as it will help women who are suffering from: fibroids, infertility, endometriosis, abnormal uterine bleeding, PCOS, POI, cervical cancer, interstitial cystitis and other female reproductive system disorder to live a healthy, happy and fruitful life without undergoing surgery.

To the author, "children are gift from God. So, don't allow any doctor to write you off that you are 'barren' because with this book, you are '**FERTILE**'.

Made in the USA
Las Vegas, NV
12 March 2024

87059837R00049